Typing Therapy Activities For ALL To Practice

How To Exercise Muscles With These 10 Computer Keyboarding Game Like Activities

Dr. Katie Canty, Ed.D.

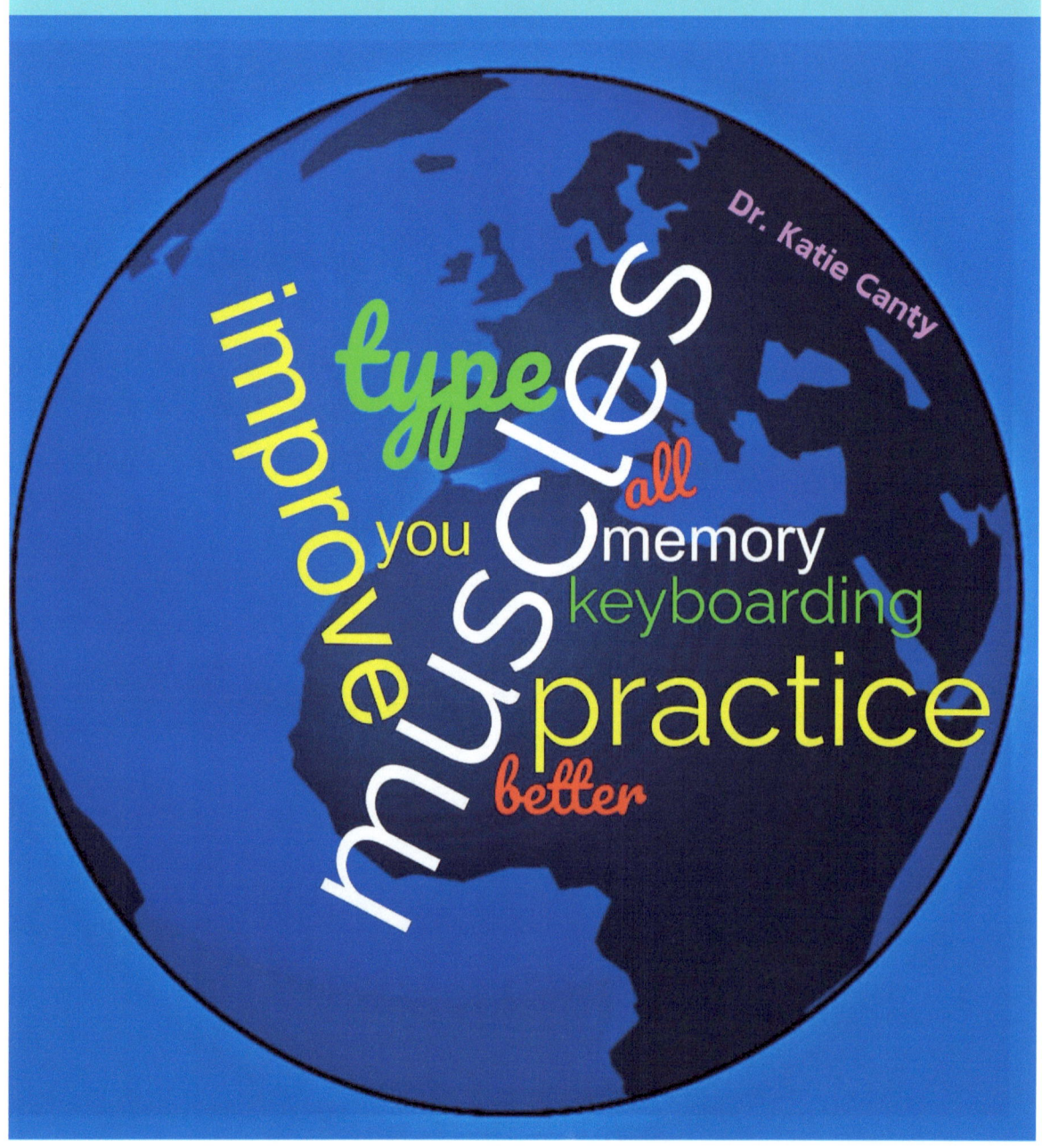

Calling all who want or need to exercise muscles:

Try these fun and engaging computer keyboarding typing exercises.

©2024

Dr. Katie Canty, Ed.D.

ISBN: 9798877248991

About

The student's socialite, wealthy parent got special permission to enroll the student in computer keyboarding class. This the teacher did not know until the class was over. The teacher was sent a "beyond thank you" message from the student's parent.

There was something else that the teacher did not know, which inspired the writing of this book. The message from the parent went on to say this.

When typing your teacher made lessons--for some unknown reason, I notice that my child who is diagnosed with a cognitive disability, is no longer disabled, especially while in your class.

The teacher did not know if this was scientifically true or not about the cognitive challenge disappearance. However, the teacher went on to write a grant to offer the course on a trial basis. And the keyboarding course became the first online course ever offered at their institution of higher learning.

This book belongs to

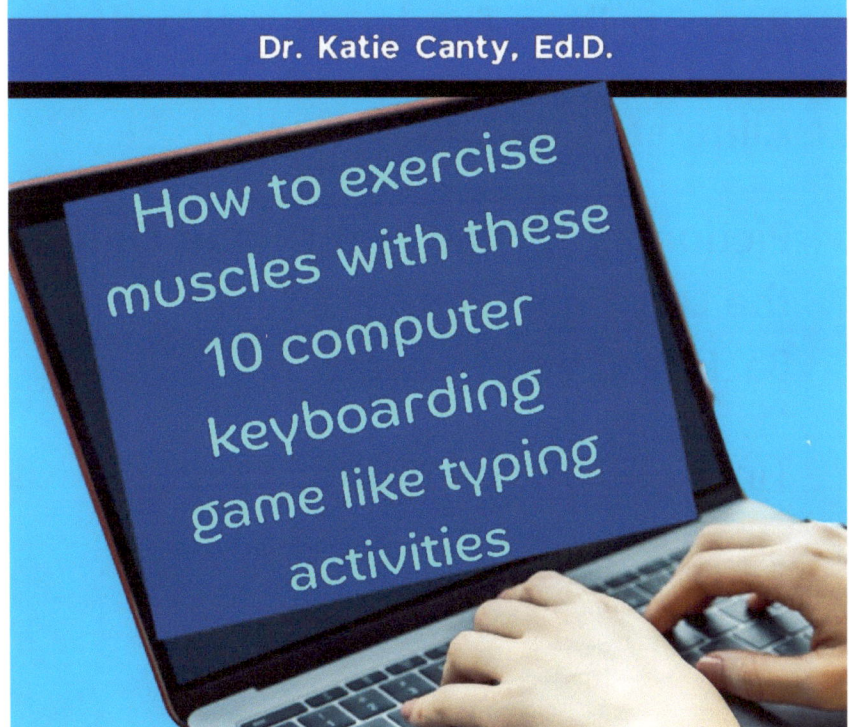

Table of Contents

Make Plans   Activity 1

My name is _____

Start date_____

Planned completion date for this book _____

Scheduled time(s) to practice is when? _____

If you have a keyboarding lessons website, the website is?

_____

The keyboarding site password is?

_____

Keyboarding teacher, tutor, helper name

_____

Email _____ Phone _____

P r e p a r e   Exercise Activity 2

1. Browse through the pages. Browsing can help you to better understand what the exercise is about and how it is designed to best help you.

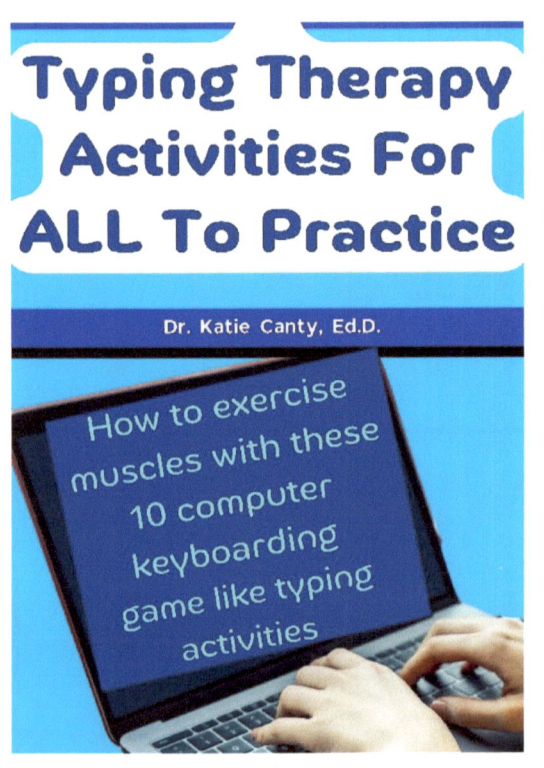

2. Gather, organize, and check your computer keyboarding typing resources. A keyboard where fingers are not cramped is recommended. Cell phones are not recommended during exercise.

3. Find a comfortable, safe, distraction-free place to type— preferably with a chair. A positive success mindset is an important resource, too.

Begin   Activity 3

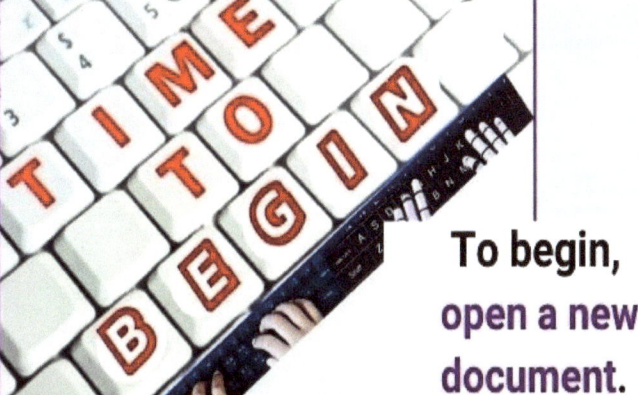

To begin, open a new document.

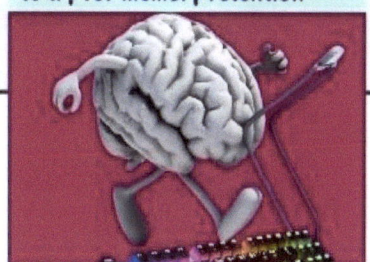

Computer keyboarding exercises to try for memory retention

Complete the positive mindset exercise activity first.

Next complete the remaining activities in any order that matches your skill level, or as assigned.

The important thing is to begin.

Open this document each time to practice an exercise activity. An example of the suggested document format is like this.

Activity No.__ Content
per exercise activity instructions

_____

_____

_____

My Success Comment

_____

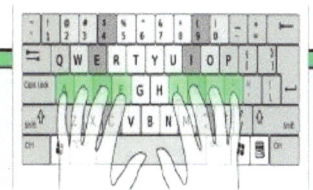

T h i n k Positive Exercise Activity 4

Your own individual
creativity is
highly encouraged.

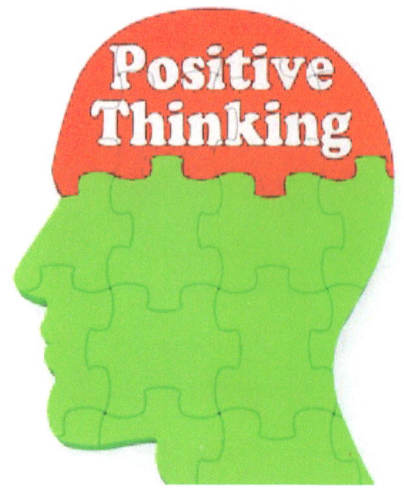

1. Think of a positive mind set quote,
affirmation, or song that you like. The idea is to motivate
yourself to complete these exercises.

2. Create a relevant image for your quote, song, or affirmation.
Type or write a comment, thought, or observation.

3. Refer to the positive mindset items as often as you need to
for motivation to type these exercise activities.

Exercise Activity 4

Positive Thinking

My Positive Thinking Creation

Instructions

1. To get an idea about what this activity involves, look at the example.

2. Open your activity practice document from Activity 3.

3. Begin and complete your Activity 4 positive thinking creation.

Hello
Techtendo 101

I gave my computer keyboard an easy to remember name--Techtendo.

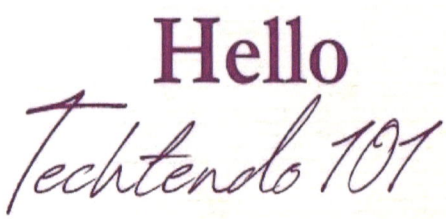

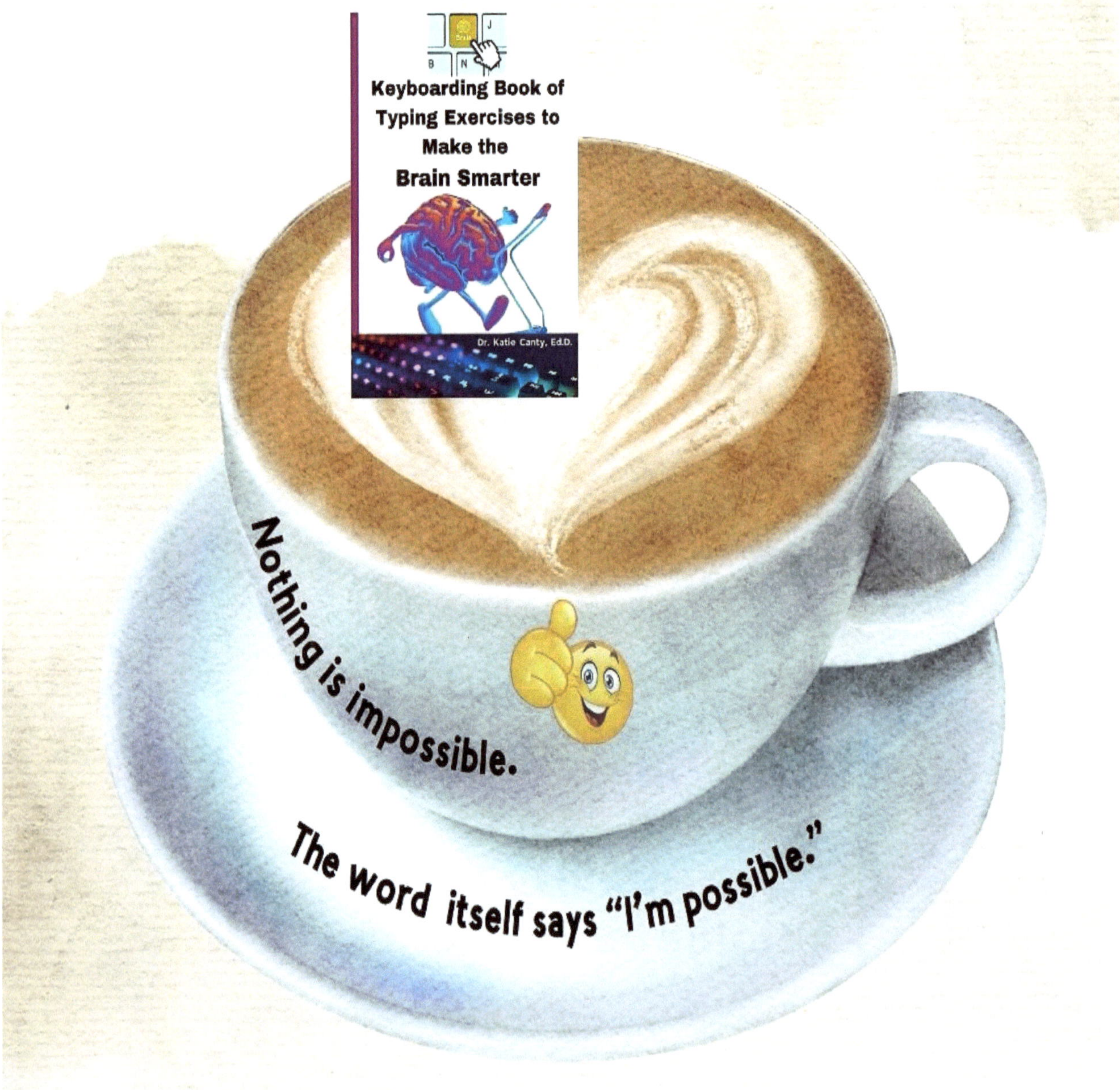

Keyboarding Book of
Typing Exercises to
Make the
Brain Smarter

Dr. Katie Canty, Ed.D.

Nothing is impossible.

The word itself says "I'm possible."

Another Example of Positive Mindset   Exercise Activity 4

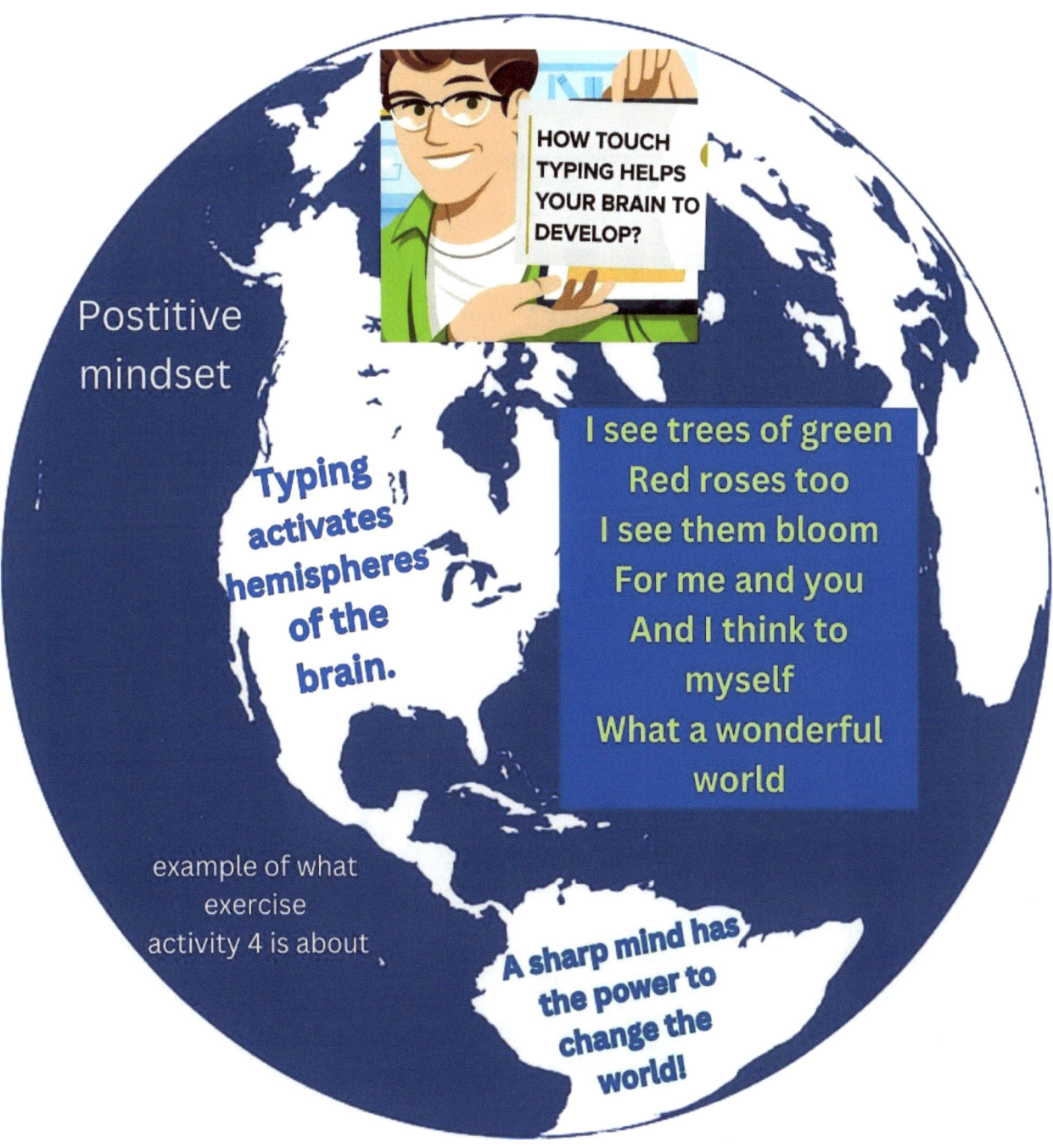

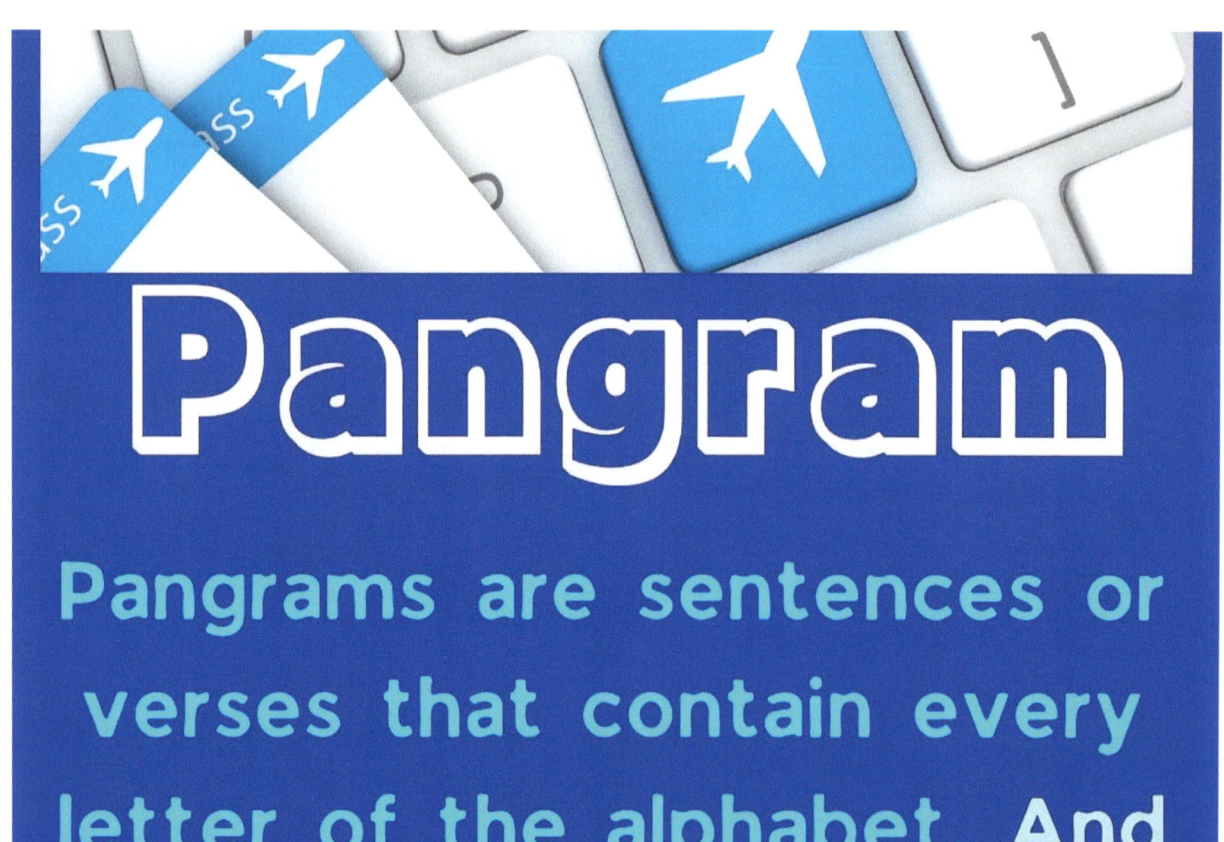

Pangram

Pangrams are sentences or verses that contain every letter of the alphabet. And they are great cognitive ability boosters.

Exercise Activity 5

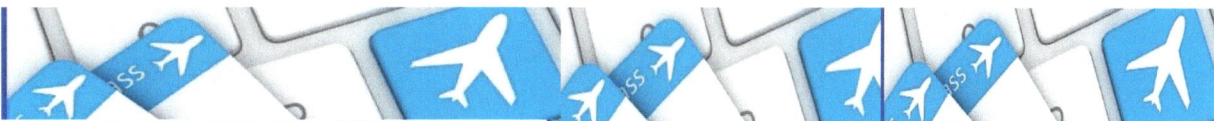

Exercise Activity 5   Pangram
Type This Sentence With All 26 Alphabets.

Instructions

•   Open your practice document to begin.

•   Practice typing the pangram line below until you can type it without an error. The ultimate goal is to type the line accurately one or more times in a minute.

Five or six big jet planes zoomed quickly by the tower.

My Success Comment

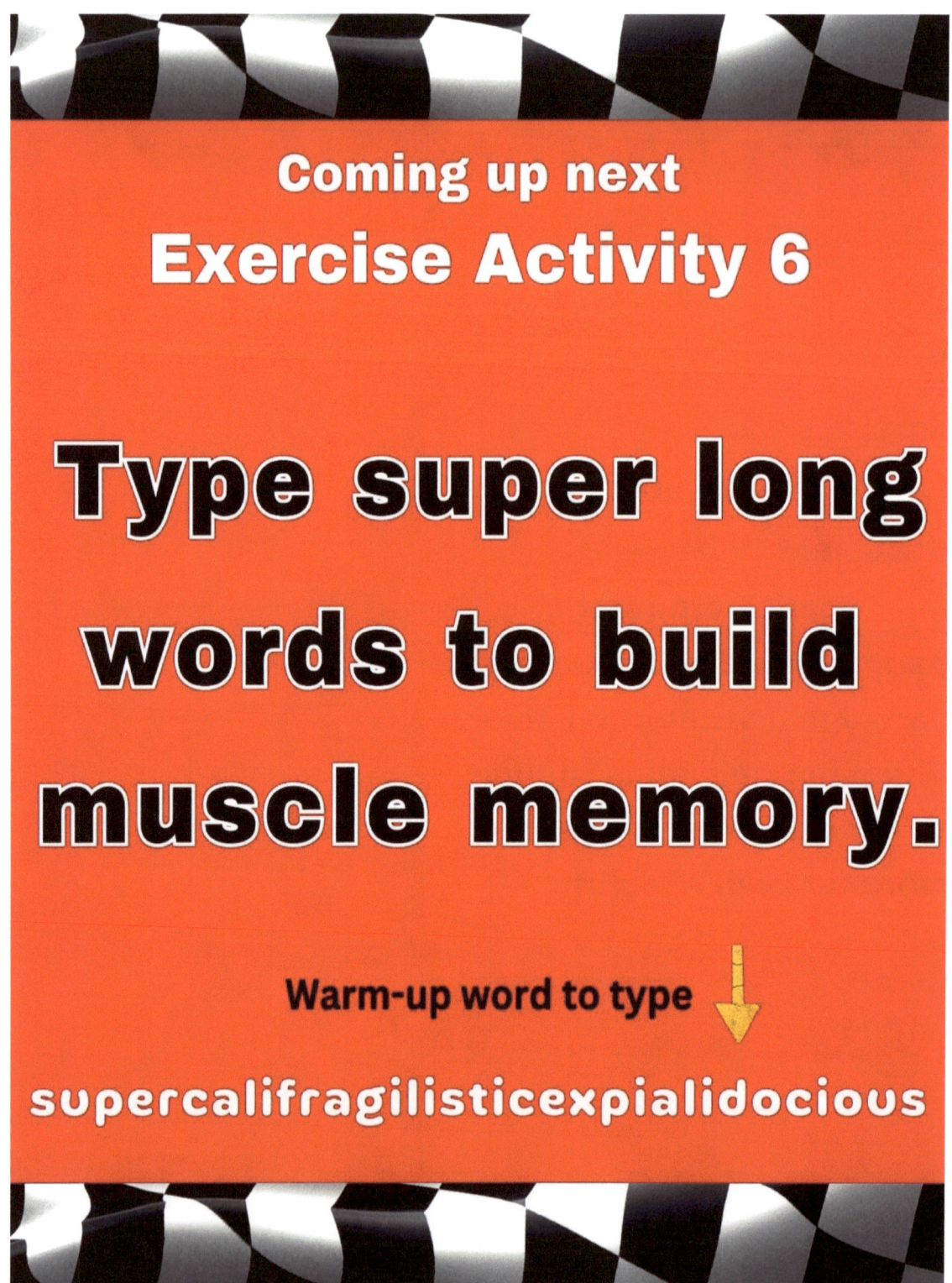

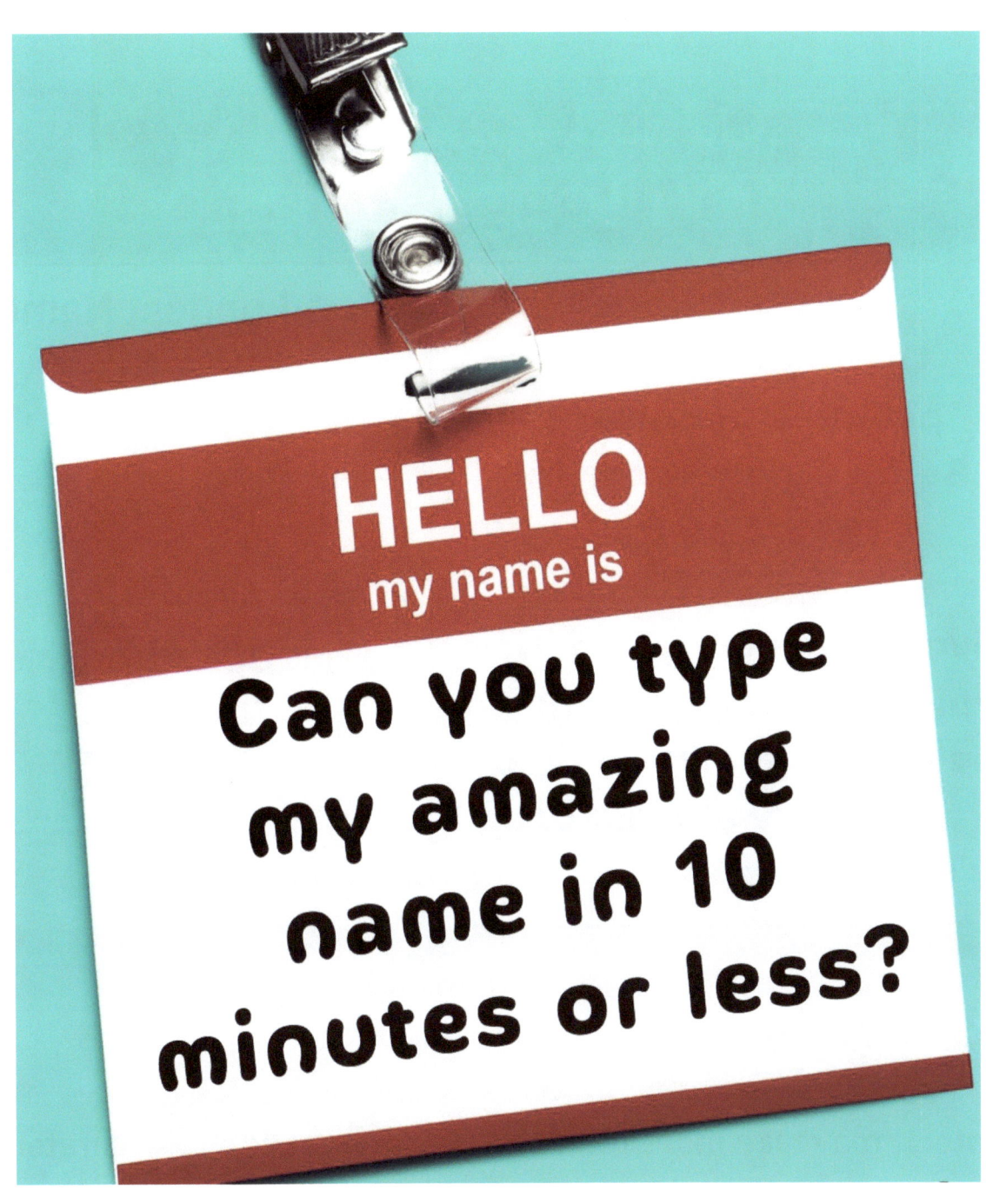

Exercise Activity 6
The Longest Name

Instructions

Open your activity practice document. Begin a new entry for Exercise 6.

Given 10 minutes, practice typing the longest name on the next page. Try to type it accurately at least one or more times.

Longest Name

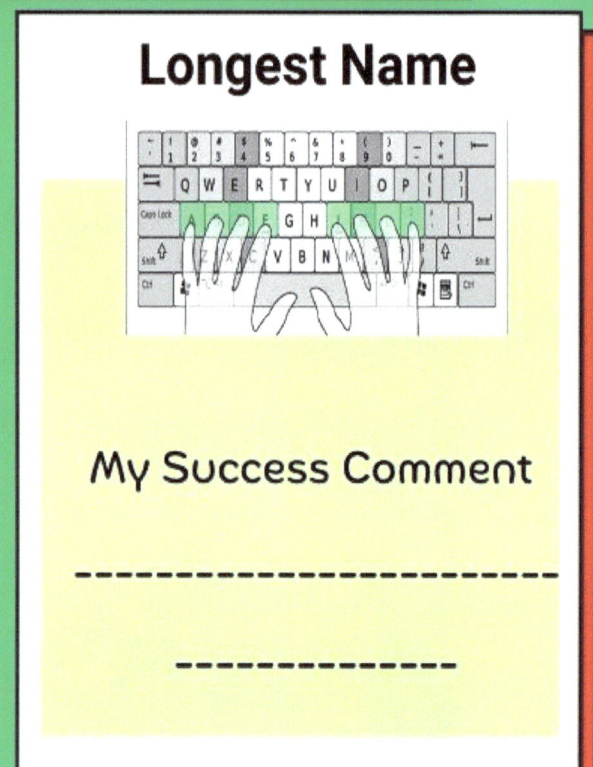

My Success Comment

Note: It may take more than one practice session to accurately complete the longest name exercise.

Exercise 6

**MaKeshaliatellyneshiaunneveshen
kescianneshaimondrischlyndasaccarnae
renquellenendrasamecashaunettethalem
eicoleshiwhalhiniveonchellecaundenesh
eaalausondrilynnejeanetrimyranaekuesa
undrilynnezekeriakenvaunetradevonneya
vondalatarneskcaevontaepreonkeinesce
ellaviavelzadawnefriendsettajerricanneles
ciajoyvaelloydietteyvettesparklenescea
undrieaquinttaekatielyaveashauwneorali
aevaekizzieshiyjuanewandaleccianneren
eitheliapreciousnesceverroneccalovelia
tyronevekacarrionnehenriettaescecleon
patrarutheliacharsalynnmeokcamonaeloies
alynnecsiannemerciadellesciaustillaparis
salondonnveshadenequamonecaalexetiozetia
quaniaenglaundneshiafrancethosharomeshaun
nehawaineakowettauandavernellchishankkarl
inaaddoneillesciachristondrafawndrealaot
relleoctavionnemiariasarahtashabnequcka
gailenaxeteshiataharadaponsadeloriakoent
escacraigneckadellanierstellavonnemyiat
angeleshiadianacorvettinagodtawadrashirl
enescekilokoneyacharrontannamyantoniaaquin
ettesequioadaurilessiaquatandamerceddiamae
bellecescajamesauwnneltomecapolotyoajohnny
aetheodoradilcyanna
Loyaanisqatsiuthawyhaiashieakhauwnne
McDougal**

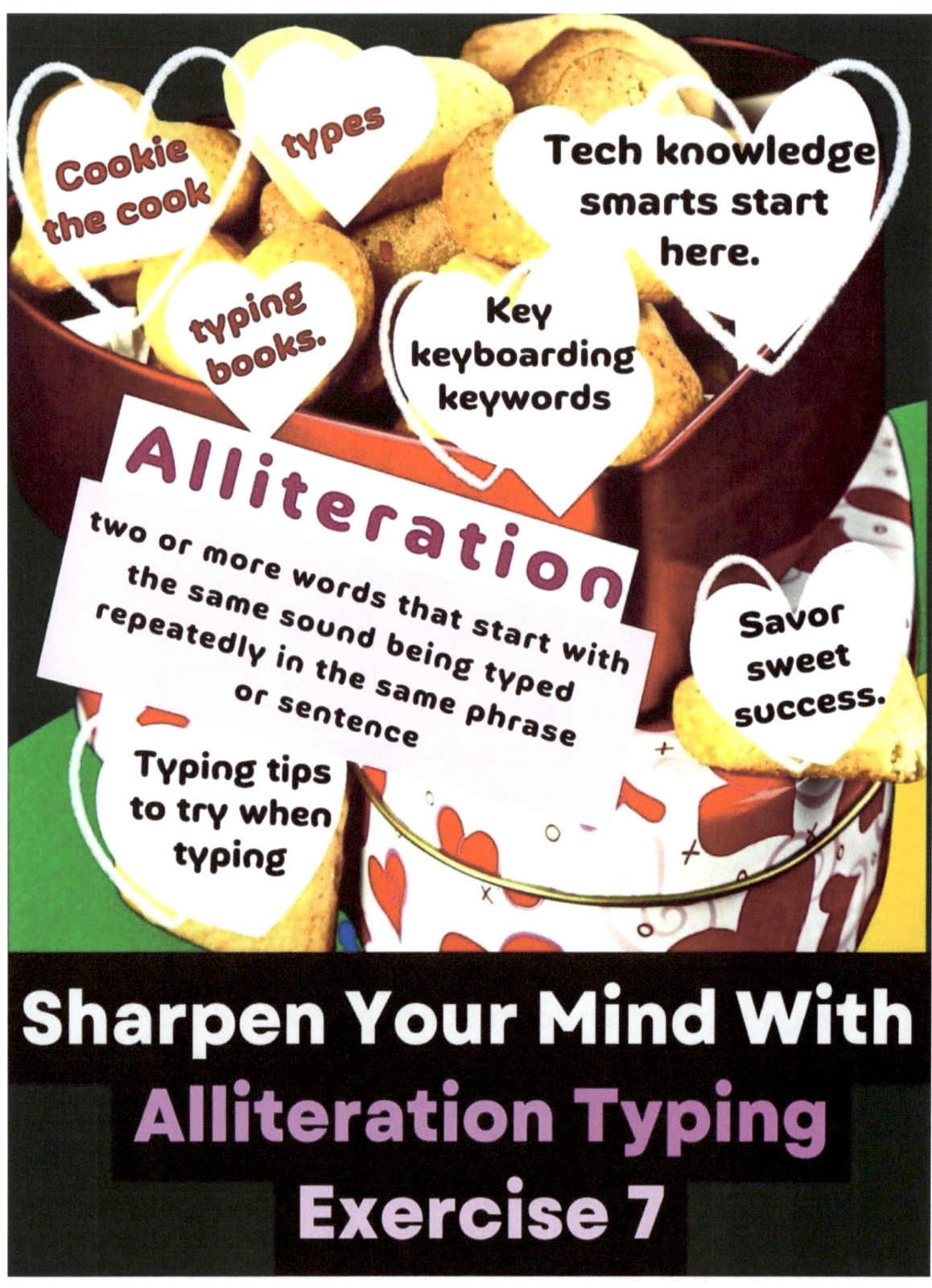

Alliterate - Type Lines A-Z.
Exercise 7

Goal
Accurately key the 26 alliteration sentences.

Objective
Try to type each alliterating sentence on the list with less than 1 error per sentence.

Instructions
Open your activity practice document. Begin to type the alliteration lines. It may take several practice sessions to accurately complete the list.

Brilliant Brain Building Alliteration Exercises

1
2
3
4
5
6
7
8
9
10
11
12
13
14
15
16
17
18
19
20
21
22
23
24
25
26

My Success Comment

	Alliterate Lines A-Z. Accurately Type Each Line.
	Exercise 7
A	Art afternoons in the park are alluring to artists.
B	Boogie Woogie Blue plays blues at the Jazzy Jazz Club.
C	Chris put the crispy coconut cookies in containers.
D	Dare to dream Dee declared with determination.
E	Everyone energetically enters the elegant eatery.
F	Friends frequently fellowship aboard this ship.
G	My great grandparent ate eight grapes every day.
H	Hound found a happy home at the campground.
I	If interested in investments, invest interest intelligently.
J	Jill and Jack journeyed to Jacksonville in a Jaguar Jeep.
K	Kindly kingdoms have kings and the kindest kind of kids.
L	Little Larry likes lemony licorice lollipops a lot.
M	Mom makes much money-making marble monuments.
N	Nine dollars buys nine new nickel-plated Ninja necklaces.
O	Orienteers occasionally offer only opposing opinions.
P	Peter Piper patiently picks purple pickled peppers.
Q	Queenie's quotes on equality quickly led to quietness.
R	Round the rugged road the rambunctious rams raced.

S	Sun shining Spring sweetly sings Summer's sweet songs.
T	Time to think thoughts that turn into timely triumphs.
U	Our university mascot is uttering unusual utterances.
V	Virtuous, vivacious veterinarians seek vacant vet jobs.
W	Wow Wee! I hear ye whispering wise words of wisdom.
X	Xan and Xanadu dress to the extreme as X-men heroes.
Y	Young yodelers on a yellow yacht yell "Yippy Ya Yah!"
Z	Zee, the zebra stripe pet, zigzags by the Zoom screen.
	Typing Therapy Activities for ALL To Practice ©2024 Katie Canty

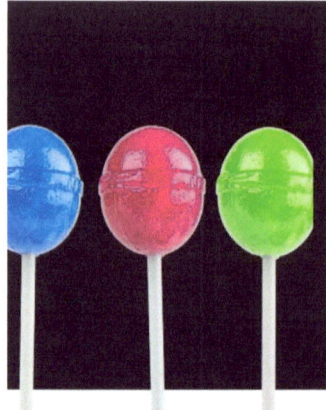

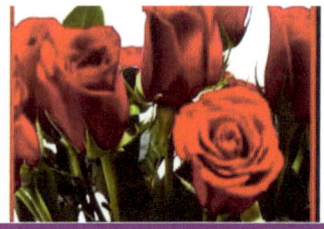

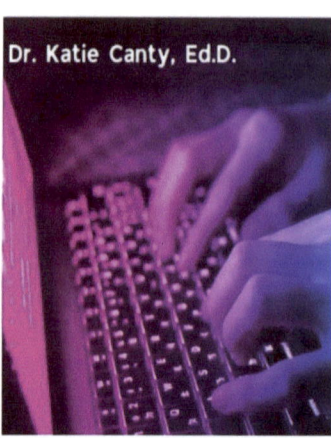

Exercise 8

Right hand Left hand

Pictionary

Type the correct answers to the 3 questions coming up. Answers are in the pictures.

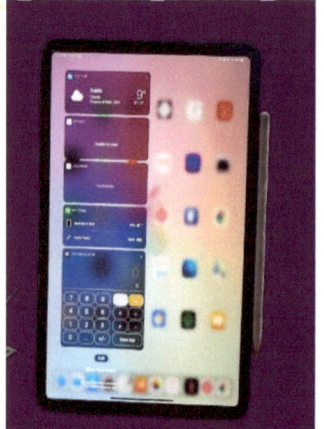

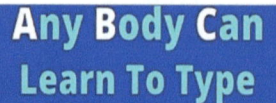

Any Body Can Learn To Type

Dr. Katie Canty, Ed.D.

New 9-Lesson Short Course

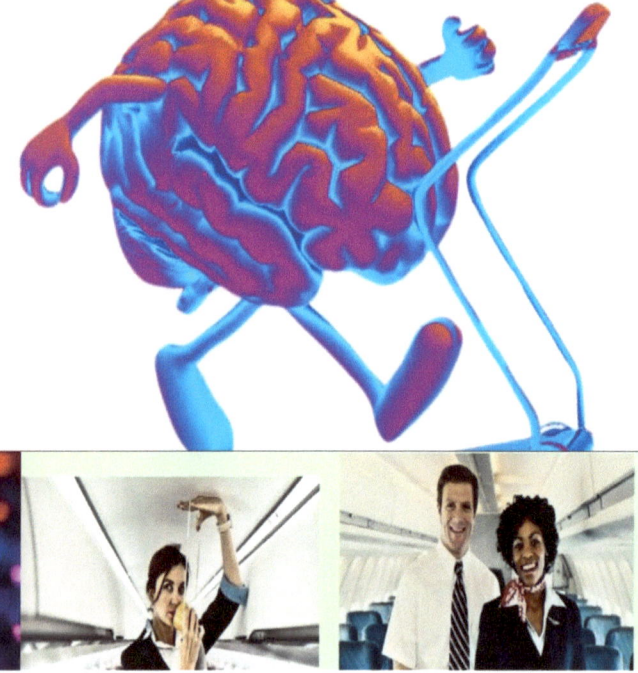

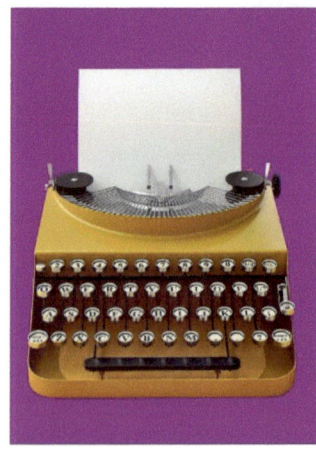

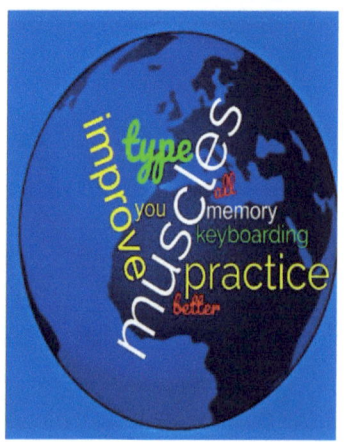

Pictionary Instructions
Exercise 8

The correct answer shows in a picture on the previous page. Based on the pictures, type the correct answer to questions 1-3 in your activity document.

1. What is the longest word that can be typed with the letter keys designated for fingers on the right hand only?
Type this word. _____

2. What is the longest word that can be typed with letter keys designated for fingers on the left hand only?
Type this word. _____

3. What is the longest word that can be typed using just letters on the second row of the keyboard only? The second row is the row under the number and symbol keys.
Type this word. _____

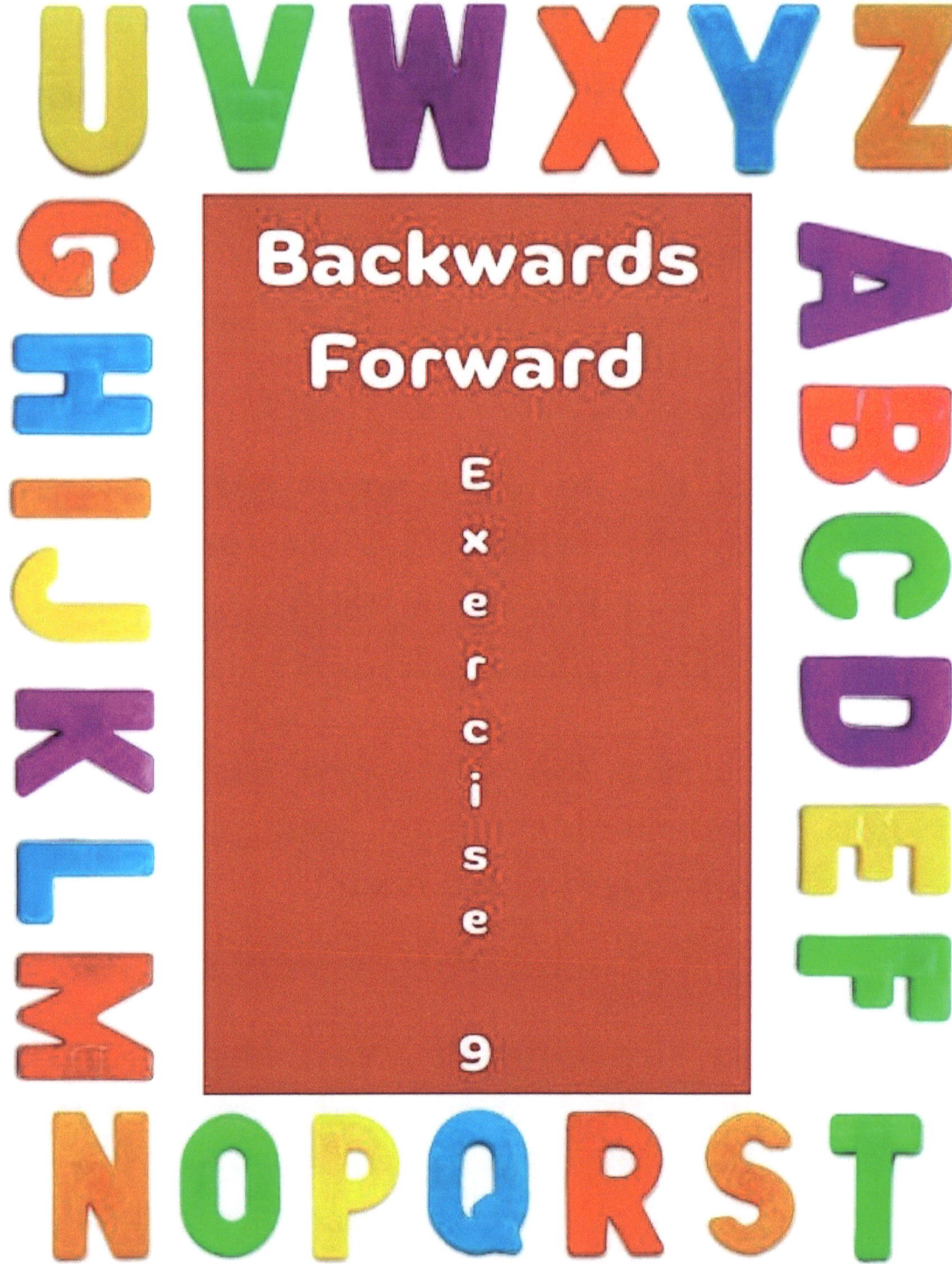

Backwards Forward

Exercise 9

Instructions   Exercise 9

1. Open your practice activity document. First, practice typing each alphabet line one or more times without being timed.

zyxwvutsrqponmlkjlhgfedcba

and

abcdefghijklmnopqrstuvwxyz

2. Next, go to a speed and accuracy alphabet typing online site that is safe and free to use for this activity. Important: If you are a school student, ask a parent or teacher first for permission to use the site(s).

We found this site at the time of writing this:
https://www.speedtypingonline.com/games/type-the-alphabet.php

3. Another suggestion is to time yourself without having to go online.

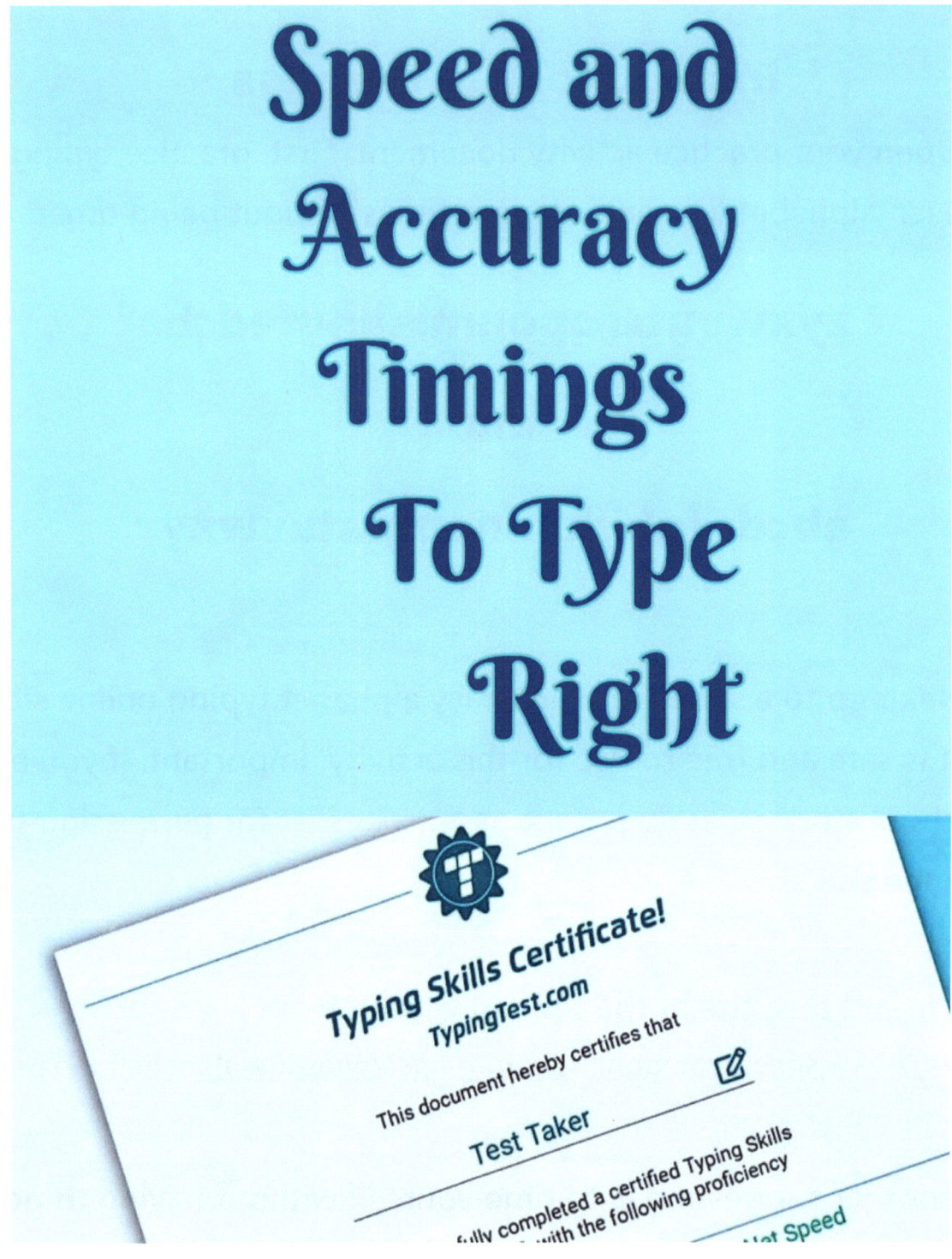

About To Finish
Speed and Accuracy
Timings   Exercise 10

Instructions

If you are a school student, first ask for parental or teacher approval to use a timed writing site. There are several free timed writing certification sites. We like typingtest.com and typing.com.

1. Go to a typing certification testing site.

2. Take a 1 minute, 3-minute, or 5-minute timed writing.

3. Save your best score results or print the results.

4. Record your best score on the certificate document on the next page.

Test Site URL _____

Typing Skills Certificate

This document hereby certifies that

_____

has successfully completed a _____ minutes certified

typing skills test on _____(date) with the

following proficiency.

Typing Speed   **Accuracy**   **Net Speed**

GWAM   Typos   WPM

Typing Therapy Activities For ALL To Practice

Dr. Katie Canty, Ed.D.

How to exercise muscles with these 10 computer keyboarding game like typing activities

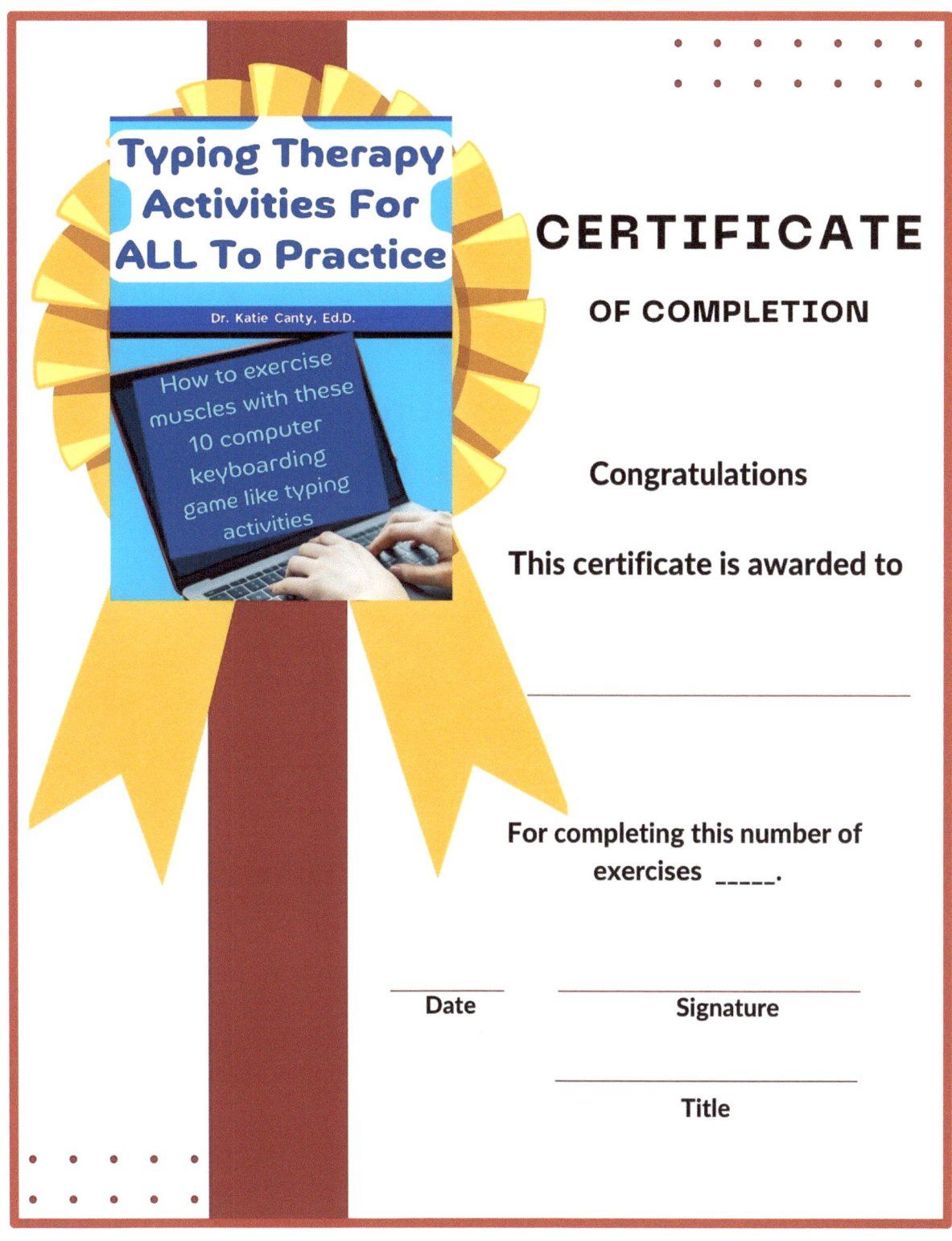

About the Author

Award winning community college educator, Dr. Katie Canty, Ed.D., helps thousands of learners to embark on successful career endeavors. To serve more learners, Dr. Canty began the non-profit organization, 1Byte Literacy, Inc. in 2004. The non-profit provides much needed tech education to elderly and disadvantaged populations.

Dr. Canty's makes her home in the South with her large family. They look forward to celebration times when Dr. Canty shows up with new game inventions and the tastiest homemade chocolate chip cookies a Mom ever baked!

Credits

canva.com

pinterest.com

pixabay.com

quora.com

timesnewsnow.com

typing.com

wordsperminute.org

youtube.com

Weekly Keyboarding Blog Task Cards on YouTube
https://www.youtube.com/channel/UCdhfJ0YZzel76onT2cbiSEw

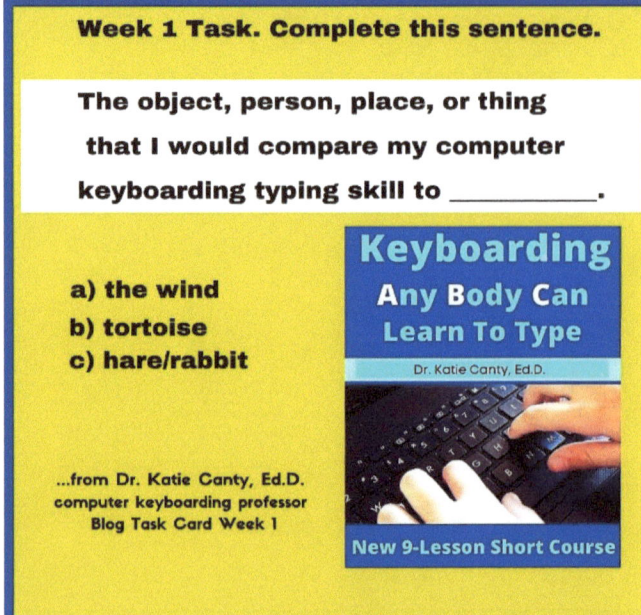

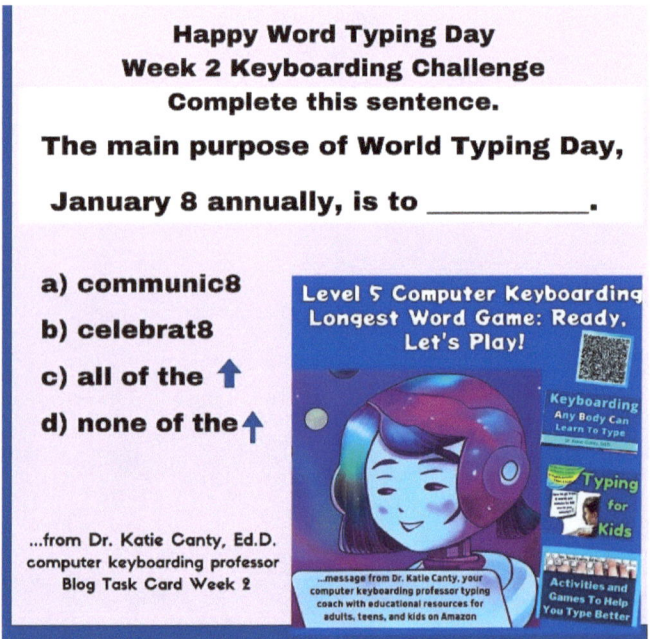

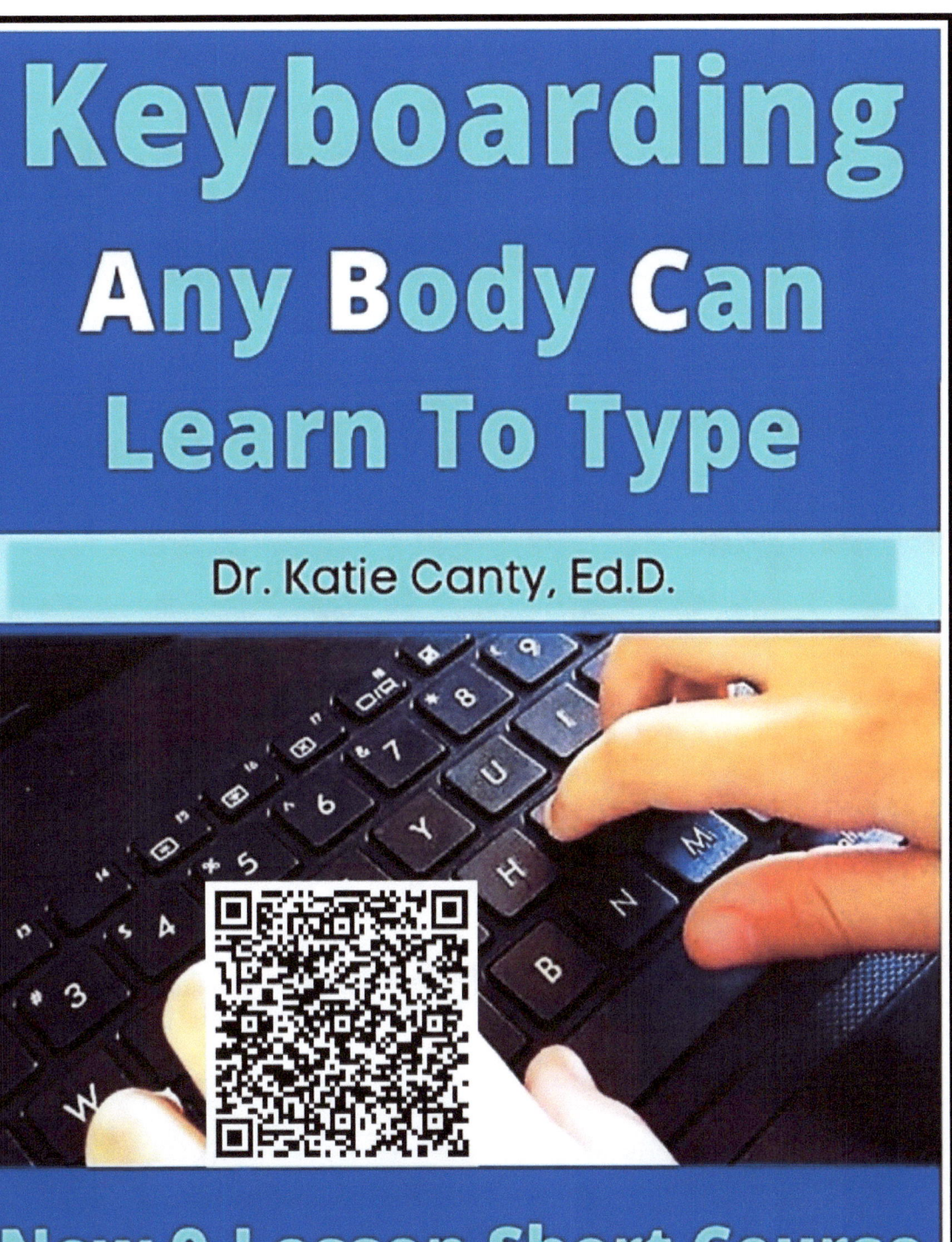

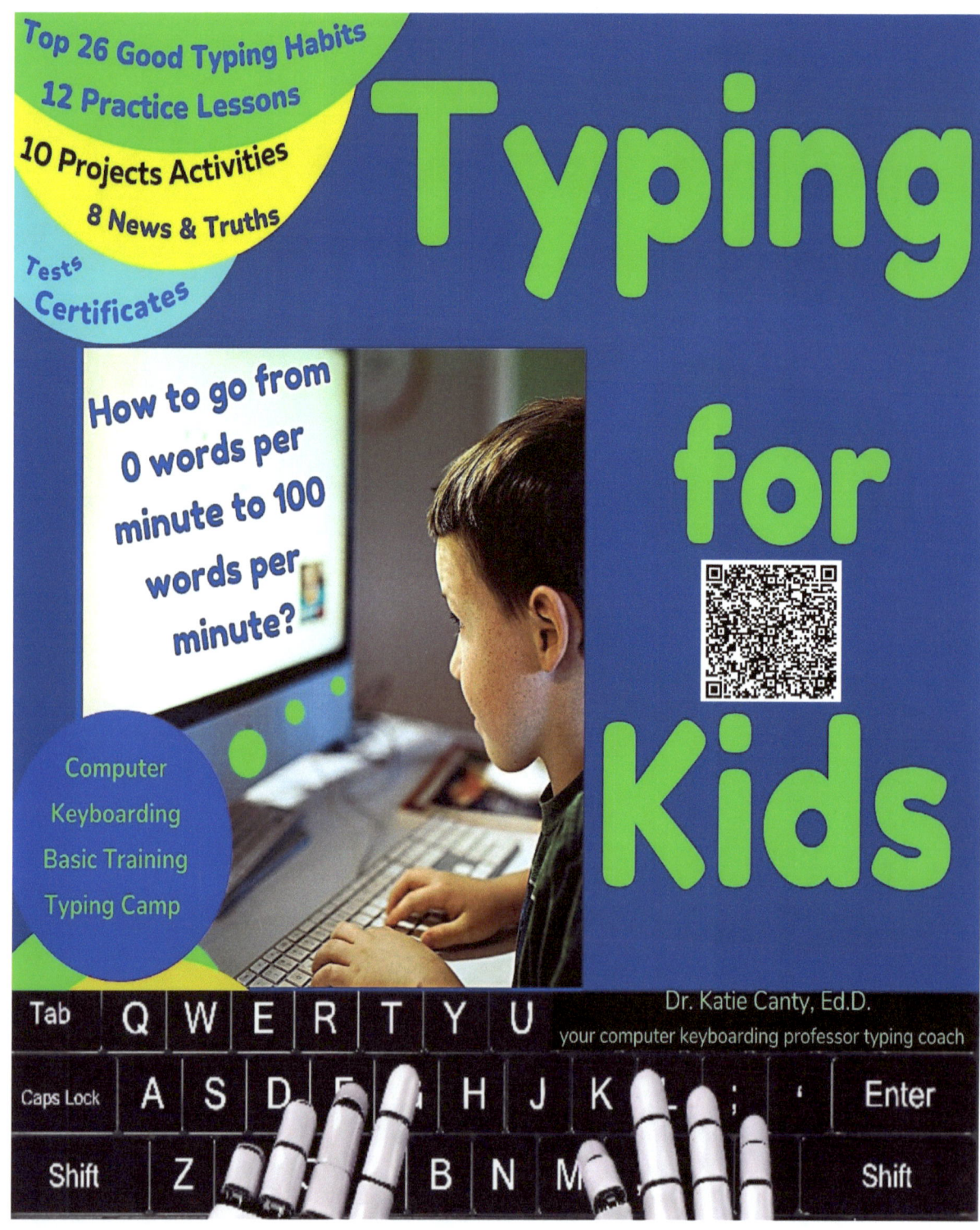

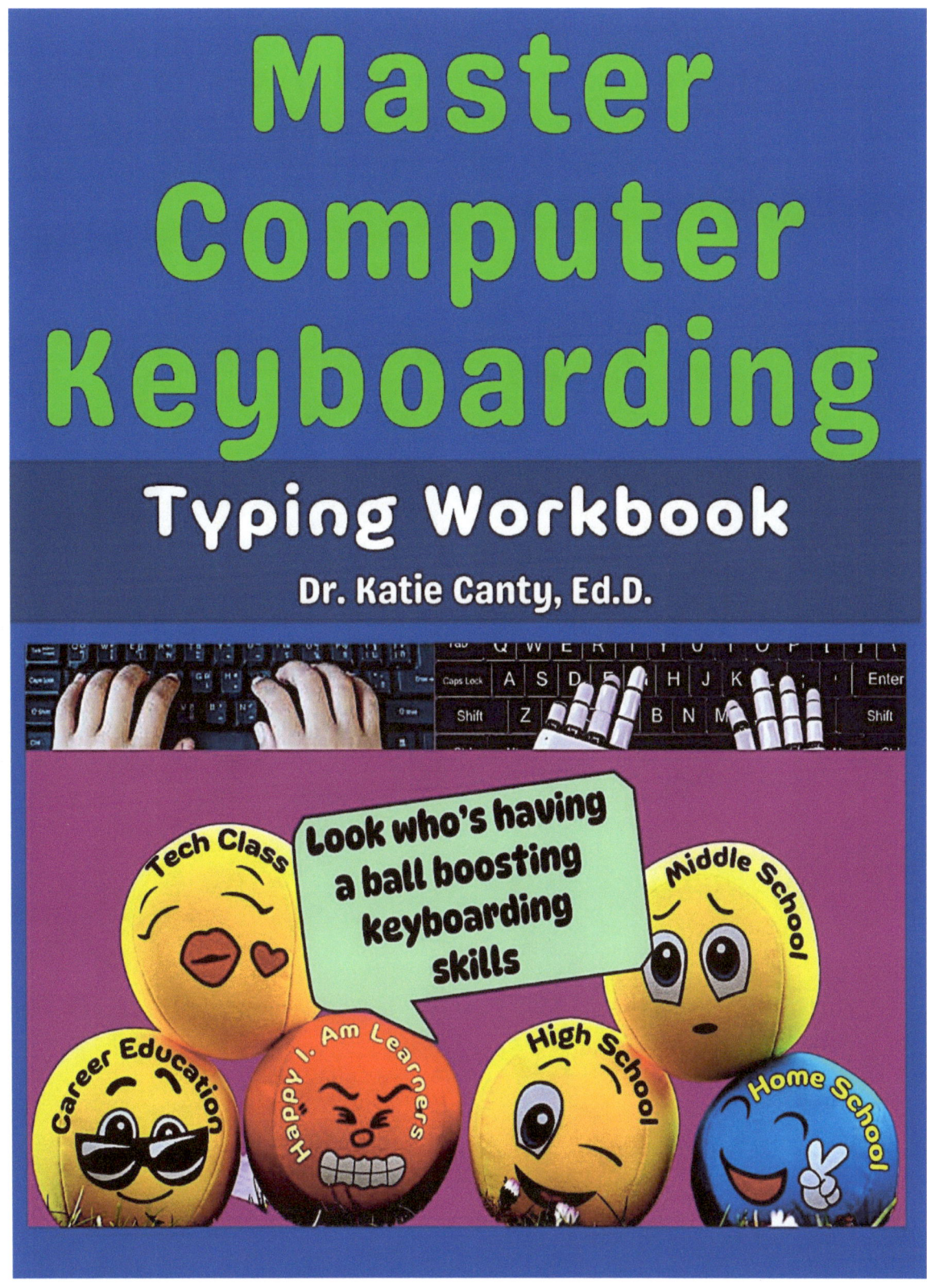

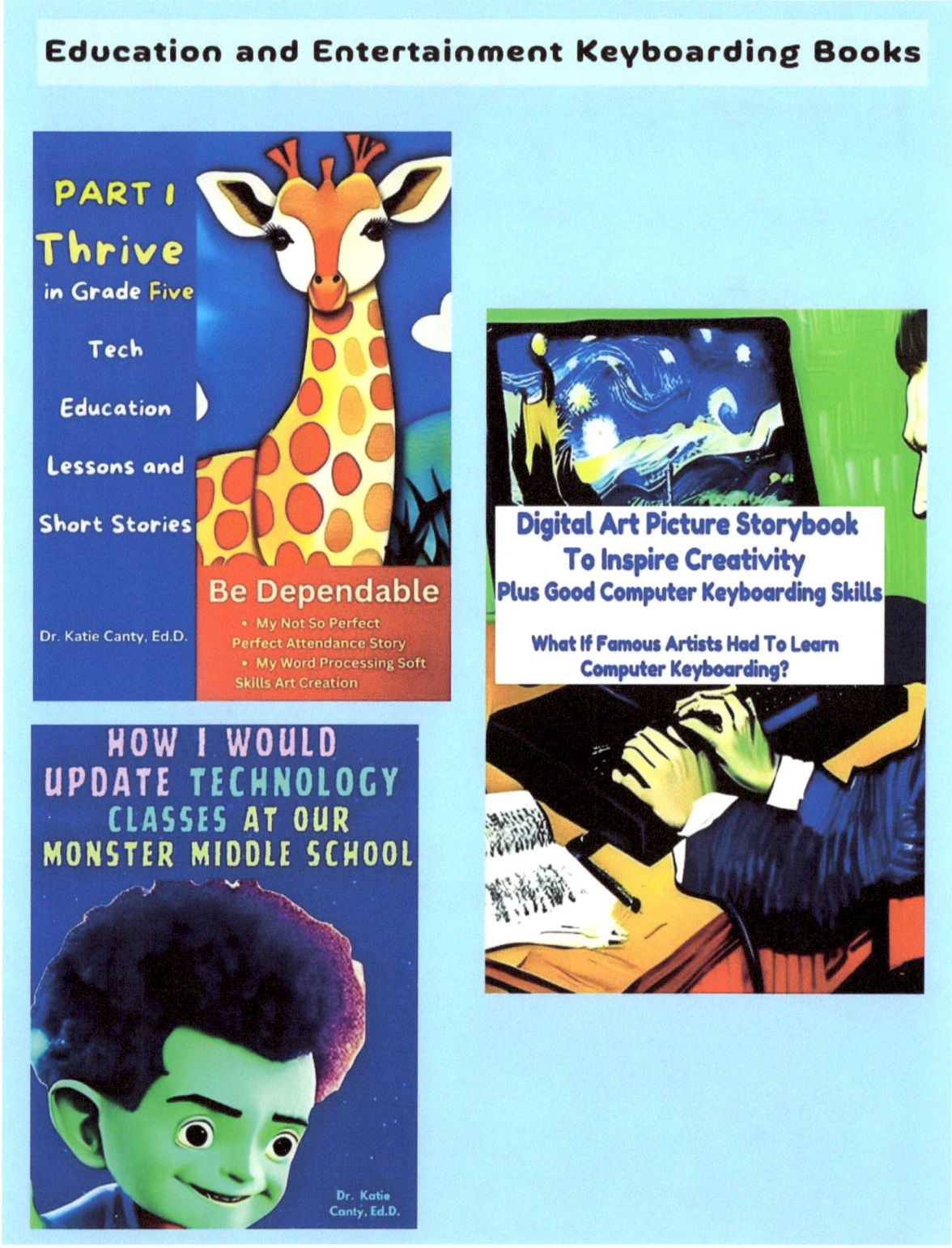

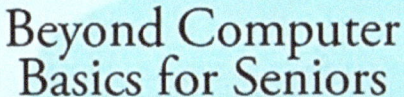

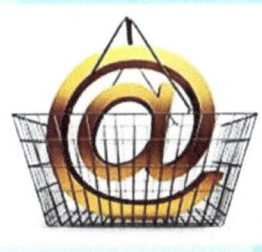

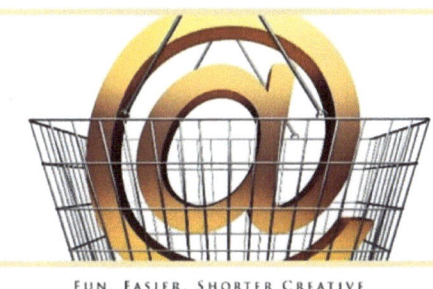

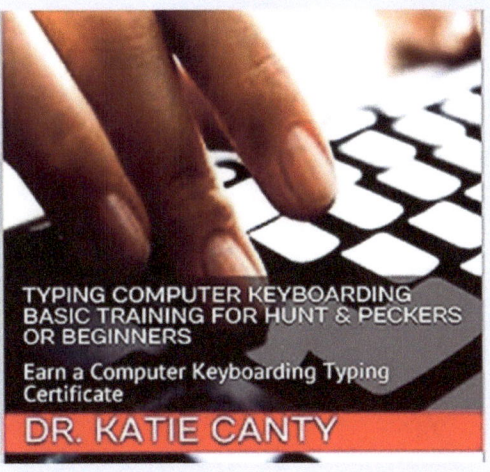

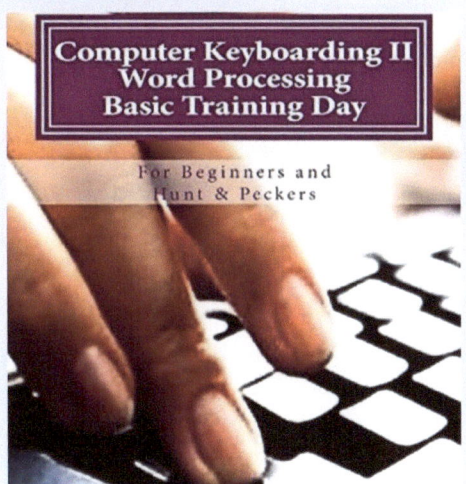

Notes

_____

_____

_____